Screens & Vision

Your Eyes in a Digital World

Guides For Eyes
Book 1

John R Martinelli MD OD FAAO

OPHTHALMIC PHYSICIAN PUBLISHING
Sharing The Fine Art of Patient Management

Contents

Medical Disclaimer

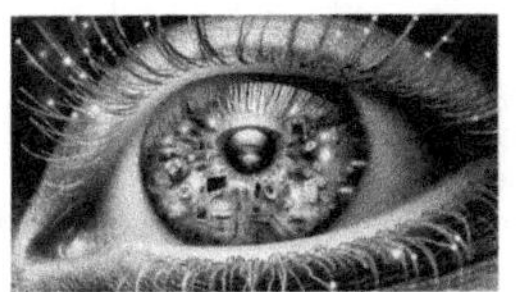

Please note the information contained within this guide is for educational purposes only. All effort has been executed to present accurate, up-to-date, reliable, complete information. The content within this guide has been derived from various sources. Please consult a licensed physician before implementing diagnostic methods and/or treatments outlined in this guide.

By reading this guide, the reader agrees that under no circumstances is the author responsible for any losses, direct or indirect, that are incurred because of the use of the information contained within this guide, including, but not limited to, errors, omissions, or inaccuracies.

Please note the information provided below is for general informational purposes. It is not intended to diagnose, treat, cure, or prevent any disease, and it should not be relied upon as a substitute for consultations with qualified healthcare professionals.

Ophthalmic Physician Publishing strives to ensure the information presented is accurate and up to date, but we make no representations or warranties of any kind, express or implied, about the completeness, accuracy, reliability, suitability, or availability with respect to the information provided. Any reliance you place on such information is strictly at your own risk.

Screens and Vision:
Your Eyes in a Digital World

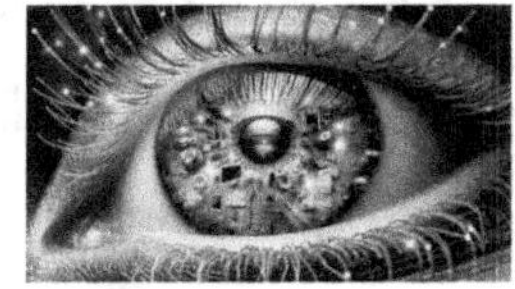

In today's digital age, our eyes are constantly exposed to screens emitting various wavelengths of light. From smartphones to laptops, these devices have become an integral part of our daily life, but they may be taking a toll on our vision. Eye strain, headaches, and disrupted sleep patterns are just a few of the issues we might face due to prolonged screen time. Understanding how light affects our eyes and overall health is key to maintaining comfortable vision in our increasingly digital world.

As we navigate our screen-dominated landscape, it's essential to know what's important for our eyes. I explore the physiology of vision in the digital era to help assess our digital habits. I'll explain environmental factors which contribute to digital eye strain, and discuss the latest in wearable technology designed to safeguard our vision. I'll also discuss workplace policies for eye health, age-related considerations for device use, and peek into the future of eye-friendly technology. By the end, you'll be better equipped with the knowledge to keep your eyes comfortable in the digital age.

Chapter 1

The Physiology of Vision in the Digital Era

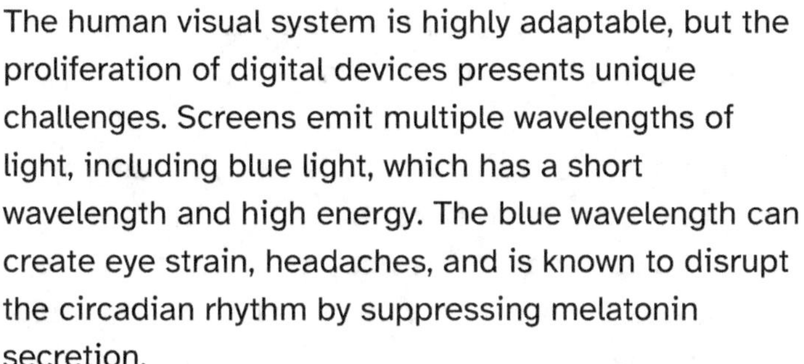

The human visual system is highly adaptable, but the proliferation of digital devices presents unique challenges. Screens emit multiple wavelengths of light, including blue light, which has a short wavelength and high energy. The blue wavelength can create eye strain, headaches, and is known to disrupt the circadian rhythm by suppressing melatonin secretion.

When viewing digital screens, our eyes must focus on pixels, which are tiny dots of light that make up the image. Unlike printed text, pixels have blurred edges, making it more difficult for our eyes to maintain focus. This can lead to digital eye strain, also known as computer vision syndrome, which affects 50-90% of computer users.

How Eyes Process Digital Images

To see digital images clearly, our eyes rapidly relax and accommodate to continuously refocus on our device's screen. This constant accommodation can lead to eye fatigue and discomfort. Additionally, digital devices are often viewed at a closer distance than printed materials, which can increase symptoms.

Accommodation and Vergence

Accommodation refers to our eye's ability to change focus from distant to near objects by altering the shape of the lens via contraction of a tiny muscle within the eye, the ciliary muscle. Vergence is the synchronized movement of both eyes in opposite directions to maintain single binocular vision. Prolonged use of digital devices can lead to accommodative and vergence disorders, contributing to digital eye strain symptoms.

Studies have shown mixed results regarding the impact of digital device use on accommodative and vergence functions. Some report reduced accommodative amplitude and facility, while others found no significant changes. However, the prevalence of accommodative and vergence disorders and symptoms among digital device users highlights the need for further research and management strategies.

The Role of the Ciliary Muscle

The ciliary muscle plays the main role in accommodation by controlling the shape of the lens by automatically contracting and relaxing. When focusing on near objects such as digital screens, the ciliary muscle contracts, allowing the lens to become more rounded. This increased curvature helps to focus light from near objects onto the retina.

Prolonged use of digital devices can lead to ciliary muscle spasms, contributing to accommodative disorders and digital eye strain symptoms. This is particularly problematic for pre-presbyopic individuals around the age of 40 who rely more heavily on their little remaining accommodative ability.

To maintain comfortable vision and reduce the risk of digital eye strain, it is essential to adopt healthy viewing habits. The 20-20-20 rule, which involves taking a 20-second break every 20 minutes to look at an object 20 feet away, can help relax the eyes and alleviate symptoms. Additionally, maintaining an appropriate viewing distance, reducing glare, and using blue light-filtering lenses may help mitigate the effects of digital device use on the visual system.

Chapter 2
Assessing Your Digital Habits

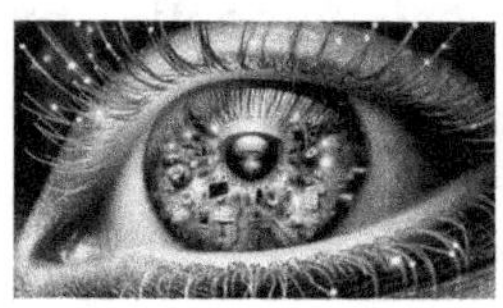

To understand the impact of digital devices on our eyes and vision, it's important to assess our screen time habits. On average, adults spend over 11 hours per day interacting with media, and 90% of adults use digital devices for two or more hours each day. This prolonged exposure to screens can lead to digital eye strain, headaches, and even disrupted sleep patterns.

Screen Time Tracking

The first step in assessing our digital habits is to track our screen time. Most smartphones and tablets have built-in features which allows monitoring daily usage. For example, Apple's Screen Time and Google's Digital Wellbeing provide detailed breakdowns of device usage, including the amount of time spent on specific apps and websites. By reviewing this data, we can gain insights into our digital habits and identify areas where we may be overusing our devices.

Identifying Harmful Patterns

Once we have tracked our screen time, look for patterns which may be creating issues. Consider the following questions:

- Do I spend long periods staring at screens without taking breaks?
- Do I use digital devices in low-light conditions or at night?
- Do I experience symptoms of digital eye strain, such as dryer eyes, blurred vision, or headaches?

If answering yes to any of these questions, it's time to make changes to our digital habits. The American Optometric Association does recommend the 20-20-20 rule: every 20 minutes, take a 20-second break and look at something 20 feet away. This simple practice can help reduce eye strain and prevent long-term discomfort and symptoms.

Setting Healthy Boundaries

In addition to taking regular breaks, it's essential to set reasonable boundaries around our digital device use. Consider implementing the following strategies:

- Establish designated screen-free times, such as during meals or before bedtime.
- Create device-free zones in your home, such as the bedroom or dining room.
- Use blue light filters or glasses to help with contrast and glare, especially in the evenings.

By setting some boundaries, we can reduce our overall screen time and minimize the impact of digital devices. Remember, while technology is an integral part of our lives, it's important to use it responsibly and prioritize our well-being.

Assessing our digital habits is the first step in helping our vision in the digital age. By tracking our screen time, identifying harmful patterns, and setting reasonable boundaries, we can reduce our risk of digital eye strain and discomfort. As we navigate the digital world, let's remember to prioritize our vision and take proactive steps.

Chapter 3

Environmental Factors Affecting Digital Eye Strain

The environment in which we use digital devices can have a significant impact on the severity of digital eye strain symptoms. Factors such as indoor lighting, outdoor light exposure, and seasonal changes can all contribute to the development or exacerbation of visual issues.

Indoor lighting plays a key role. Fluorescent lighting has been known to spur eyestrain, and incandescent light can also trigger symptoms. To stay most comfortable, it is recommended to position desks at right angles to a window or off to the side, rather than facing into a window. Overhead ceiling lights should also be behind a desk or off to the side and not visible in peripheral vision when working at a desk. Glare from direct and indirect light sources, such as windows, desk lamps, and ceiling lights, can slow down reading speed. Therefore, it's essential to set up work and study spaces free of direct light sources in the field of view.

Outdoor light exposure is another significant factor. Spending time outdoors has been shown to have a protective effect against myopia development and progression in children and teenagers. This benefit appears to be due to the brightness of outdoor light, which can be 500 times brighter than indoors, even when under shade and wearing a hat and sunglasses. However, it's important to practice sun safety when spending time outdoors, as excessive sun exposure can lead to eye diseases in later life, such as eye surface disorders, cataract, and age-related macular degeneration.

Seasonal changes can also impact our eyes and contribute digital eye strain. In the winter months, there is far less natural light, requiring our eyes to work extra hard to complete tasks, even when artificial light is present. Additionally, the transition from daylight saving time to standard time can throw off sleep patterns, which is impactful due to the direct correlation between the quality of sleep and visual symptoms. Winter weather also means decreased moisture levels, leading to dryer eyes. The combination of brisk outdoor air and increased indoor heating can lead to dryness, including the skin, lips, lids, and surface of the eyes. The best way to combat eye dryness in the winter is to use over-the-counter artificial tears regularly and hydrate as much as possible.

Remember environmental factors such as indoor lighting, outdoor light exposure, and seasonal changes can all contribute to the development or exacerbation of digital eye discomfort. By being aware of these factors and taking appropriate measures, such as setting up work and study spaces free of direct light sources, spending time outdoors while practicing sun safety, and using artificial tears and hydrating during the winter months, we will minimize the risk of uncomfortable symptoms.

Chapter 4
Wearable Technology and Vision

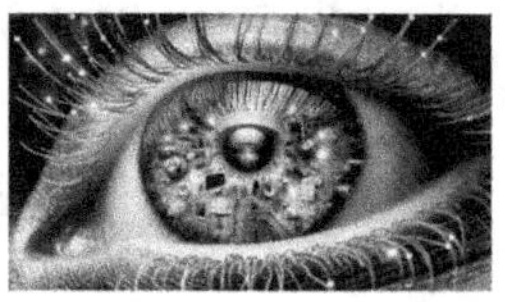

As technology advances, wearable devices are becoming increasingly popular in the digital age. These devices, such as smart glasses, VR headsets, and contact lenses with digital displays, offer unique experiences but also raise concerns about their impact on our eyes.

Smart glasses, like the Meta Ray-Ban glasses, allow users to make calls, listen to music, and capture photos and videos that can even be live-streamed on social media. These glasses also feature a digital assistant powered by artificial intelligence. While stylish and functional, it's essential to consider the potential effects of prolonged use on visual comfort and also clarity.

Virtual reality (VR) headsets provide immersive experiences by projecting images directly onto our eyes, creating a stereoscopic effect which gives the illusion of depth. However, the close proximity of these devices has led us to question the potential negative effects, especially when used for extended periods. Visual discomfort and blur, headaches, and disrupted sleep patterns are some of the concerns now associated with VR use. While permanent VR eye damage is not a major concern at present, more research is needed to fully understand the long-term effects on eyes and vision.

To minimize the risk of visual discomfort while using VR, it's recommended to take frequent breaks, follow the 20-20-20 rule (taking a 20-second break every 20 minutes to look at an object 20 feet away), and adjust the headset for a comfortable fit. Paying attention to our body and limiting VR session times according to personal comfort are also important strategies for using these devices.

Contact lenses with digital displays are an emerging technology which combines the convenience of contact lenses with the functionality of smart devices. Companies like Mojo Vision are developing smart contact lenses which feature high-resolution microLED displays, wireless data transfer, and eye-tracking capabilities.

These lenses are designed to project information directly onto the back of our eye, the retina, providing a discreet and hands-free experience. However, as with any new technology, we must consider the potential impact on physical eye health. Mojo Vision is currently working closely with the FDA to ensure the safety and efficacy of their smart contact lenses before making them available to the public.

While wearable technology offers exciting possibilities for enhancing our digital experiences, it's essential to also prioritize physical eye health with certain technologies as well as comfort. As these devices become more commonplace, remember to follow guidelines for safe use, take regular breaks, and consult with your eye care professional to monitor potential effects on vision. By staying informed and proactive, you can enjoy the benefits of wearable technology while minimizing the risk of digital eye strain and other eye-related issues.

Chapter 5

Workplace Policies for Eye Health

As the digital landscape continues to shape our work environments, it's important for employers to prioritize eye health and vision by implementing policies which protect their employees' eyes. By adopting eye-friendly practices, conducting ergonomic assessments, and educating employees on digital eye strain, companies can create a safer and more productive workplace.

Implementing Eye-Friendly Practices

Simple, everyday adjustments can significantly minimize visual issues and symptoms in the workplace, whether in a traditional office or at home. To mitigate digital eye strain, place computer monitors at the right height and distance from the eyes, about 4-5 inches below eye level and 20-28 inches away. Encouraging frequent screen breaks, and blinking often to moisten and refresh the eyes.

Adjusting screen brightness to match ambient light levels and choosing easy-to-read font styles can also be helpful.

Cutting glare is another essential aspect of creating an eye-friendly workspace. Positioning computer screens and workspaces to prevent glare, and wall coverings which don't create reflections. Installing window films, blinds, or sheer curtains can help control light, while anti-glare screens for monitors can decrease reflected light.

Regulating the environment is also key. For example, a flexible office space allowing employees and staff to move around to avoid dry moving air blowing on their eyes or faces. Adjusting the thermostat and air conditioner direction, as well as using air filters and humidifiers, can minimize discomfort and symptoms.

Employee Education on Digital Eye Strain

Educating about digital eye strain should be policy for maintaining eye health and comfort in the workplace. Digital eye strain occurs when spending extended periods staring at screens, triggering issues like burning and watering, blurred vision, headaches, neck and shoulder pain, difficulty focusing, and sensitivity to light.

Promoting employee education by providing resources on digital eye strain, such as informational posters, emails, or workshops should be the norm.

Encouraging regular eye exams is also imperative, as vision and eye health change gradually during daily life activities, and the best way to identify these changes is through annual check-ups.

By implementing eye-friendly practices, conducting ergonomic assessments, and educating on digital eye strain, companies can create a workplace which prioritizes eye health, vision, and overall well-being. As the digital age continues to shape our work environments, it's essential for employers to adapt and provide the necessary support to protect their employees in terms of not only eye safety, but also vision.

Chapter 6
Age-Related Considerations for Digital Device Use

As technology becomes increasingly integrated into our daily lives, it's important to consider age-related factors which can influence digital device use and its impact on eyes and vision. From children to seniors, each age group faces unique challenges and considerations when it comes to screen time.

Children and Screen time

Children are spending more time than ever in front of screens, which can have a significant impact on their eyes and visual development. Prolonged exposure to blue light from digital devices has been linked to blurred vision, headaches, and disrupted sleep patterns. To minimize these symptoms, parents should set realistic limits on screen time and encourage healthy habits, such as taking frequent breaks and maintaining an appropriate viewing distance.

Studies have also found children who spend more time indoors are more likely to develop nearsightedness (myopia). Exposure to natural daylight plays an important role in normal eye and visual development, so it's recommended for children to spend more time outdoors engaging in physical activities instead of in front of a screen.

Adult Vision Changes

As adults age, their vision naturally undergoes changes which can affect their ability to use digital devices comfortably. Presbyopia, a natural aging process which makes it difficult to focus on close-up objects and reading, typically begins to develop in the early to mid-40s. This can make it challenging to read small text on screens or work on computers for extended periods.

To accommodate these changes, adults may need to adjust their screen settings, such as increasing font size or brightness, or invest in prescription computer glasses. Screen magnifiers are also available. Most importantly, regular eye exams are essential and always recommended first for detecting and addressing age-related eye disorders or vision problems.

Seniors and Technology Adaptation

Older adults face several barriers when it comes to adapting to new technologies, including physical limitations, cognitive changes, and a lack of familiarity with digital devices. Visual impairments, such as age-related macular degeneration and cataracts, can make it difficult for seniors to read screens or navigate complex interfaces.

To overcome these challenges, technology designed for seniors can prioritize user-friendly interfaces, simple functions, and accessibility features. Training and support is also important and can be available for helping older adults build confidence and competence with digital devices.

Assistive technologies, such as screen readers, voice-activated controls, and large-print keyboards, can help seniors with significant visual or physical impairments access the benefits of technology. By addressing the unique needs and challenges of older adults, we can ensure everyone has the opportunity to engage with digital devices properly and effectively.

Age-related considerations are a priority in how individuals interact with digital devices and the potential impact on their visual capacity. By understanding these factors and implementing appropriate strategies, appropriate digital habits will support new visual demands in an increasingly digital world.

Chapter 7

Future Trends in Eye-Friendly Technology

As technology continues to evolve, we can expect to see significant advancements in eye-friendly solutions which prioritize our visual demands in the digital age. From AI-driven eye care to innovative display technologies and personalized vision protection, the future holds promising developments which will transform the way you and I interact with devices and screens.

AI is poised to revolutionize eye care by automating tasks that require clinical expertise, particularly in ophthalmological diagnoses. Deep learning algorithms have demonstrated expert-level accuracy in detecting various eye conditions, such as diabetic retinopathy, age-related macular degeneration, and glaucoma, using retinal photography and optical coherence tomography. These AI systems could facilitate a reorientation of eye health service provisions, centering it on primary care and reducing the burden on surgical specialists.

In addition to AI, advancements in display technology will play a significant role in promoting eye-friendly digital experiences. Emerging technologies like 6G telecommunications and the Internet of Things (IoT) will continue to enhance the development of intelligent wearable devices for health monitoring. These devices will seamlessly integrate with our digital ecosystem, actually providing real-time data on our eye health.

Personalized vision protection will also become increasingly important in the future. As big data is generated and processed at a personal level, AI algorithms can leverage this information to create customized eye care solutions tailored to your unique needs. For example, your digital devices could automatically adapt display settings based on your age, visual acuity, and daily screen time habits, ensuring an optimal viewing experience minimizing the chance of visual discomfort.

Moreover, advancements in lens technology will offer enhanced protection against blue light and glare. Smart glasses and even contact lenses with digital displays will incorporate advanced features like anti-fog coatings, photochromic technology, and embedded sensors to monitor our eyes and visual function in real-time. These innovations will not only safeguard our vision but also provide a more comfortable and immersive digital experience.

However, the adoption of these eye-friendly technologies will require addressing several challenges. Regulatory barriers, health care infrastructural limitations, financial costs, cybersecurity risks, and ethical concerns are among the hurdles which will need to be overcome. Collaborative efforts between researchers, innovators, policymakers, and medical providers will be essential to navigate these challenges and ensure responsible and equitable implementation of eye-friendly solutions.

As we look towards the future, we can anticipate a digital landscape which prioritizes our eye health and well-being. With AI-driven eye care, cutting-edge display technologies, and personalized vision solutions, we'll be empowered to embrace the digital world without compromising our visual capacity. By staying informed about these advancements and advocating for their responsible deployment, we can play an active role in shaping a future where technology and eye care go hand in hand.

Chapter 8
Finally...

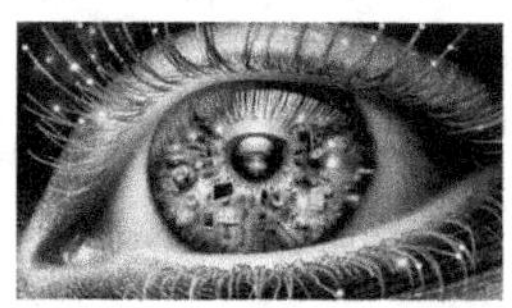

It's clear the impact of our devices and screens on our eyes has become a major aspect of modern life. From understanding the physiology of vision to assessing our digital habits and exploring workplace policies, my goal is to introduce you to current topics in a short and simple guide. The future truly does hold promise with eye-friendly technologies and personalized solutions continuing to emerge, augmenting our daily lives.

For now, remember to implement the strategies discussed, such as following the 20-20-20 rule and creating ergonomic workspaces. You will likely minimize visual discomfort and symptoms associated with prolonged screen time. Finally, as we move forward in this digital age, also remember to stay current and informed about the latest developments in eye care, vision technology, and eye health. It's moving very very fast...

Chapter 9
FAQ's

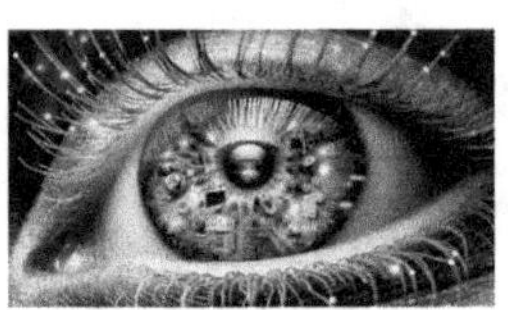

1. What are the key takeaways from this guide for maintaining eye health in the digital age?

• The guide emphasizes the importance of managing screen time, adopting ergonomic practices, using blue light filters, and taking regular breaks to prevent digital eye strain. It also highlights the significance of staying informed about the latest advancements in eye-friendly technology.

2. How can I implement the 20-20-20 rule effectively in my daily routine?

• Set a timer on your computer or smartphone to remind you every 20 minutes. During the break, look at an object that is at least 20 feet away for 20 seconds. This practice helps reduce eye strain and refreshes your eyes.

3. What types of blue light filters are available, and how do I choose the right one?

• Blue light filters come in various forms, including screen protectors, computer glasses, and software applications. Choose a filter based on your specific needs, such as the type of device you use most frequently and the level of blue light filtering required.

4. **Are there specific exercises I can do to strengthen my eye muscles?**

• Yes, exercises like focusing on a distant object, following the 20-20-20 rule, and practicing eye movements (such as looking left to right and up and down) can help maintain eye muscle flexibility and reduce strain.

5. **How can I reduce glare and improve lighting in my workspace?**

• Position your screen to minimize glare from windows and overhead lights. Use adjustable blinds or curtains to control natural light, and consider using a desk lamp with adjustable brightness. Anti-glare screen protectors can also be helpful.

6. **What should I do if I experience persistent symptoms of digital eye strain despite following the guide's advice?**

• If symptoms persist, it's important to consult an eye care professional. They can perform a comprehensive eye examination to rule out underlying conditions and recommend personalized treatments or adjustments.

7. How can parents ensure their children are developing healthy digital habits?

• Encourage regular breaks, outdoor play, and limit screen time according to age-appropriate guidelines. Create screen-free zones in the home and model healthy digital habits yourself.

8. What are some emerging technologies that could benefit my eye health?

• Emerging technologies include smart glasses with blue light filtering, advanced VR headsets designed for reduced eye strain, and smart contact lenses with digital displays. Stay updated on new developments and consider incorporating these into your digital routine.

9. How can I keep up with the latest research and developments in eye health?

• Subscribe to reputable eye health newsletters, follow professional organizations like the American Academy of Optometry and the American Medical Association, and stay connected with eye care professionals.

10. What additional resources or guides do you recommend for further reading on eye health?

• Some recommended resources include "Blue Light Exposed: Understanding the Impact of Blue Light on Our Lives" by Dr. Edward Karlik and "Digital Eye

Strain: A Clinical Guide" by Dr. Larry Abel. Additionally, websites like the American Optometric Association (AOA) and the American Academy of Ophthalmology (AAO) offer valuable information and updates.

Chapter 10
Glossary

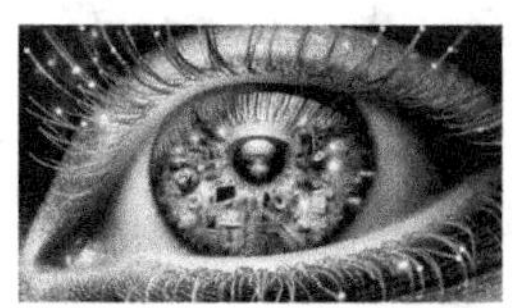

Accommodation

The eye's ability to change focus from distant to near objects by altering the shape of the lens. This process is controlled by the ciliary muscle.

Blue Light

A type of light with a short wavelength and high energy emitted by digital screens, which can contribute to eye strain and disrupt sleep patterns.

Ciliary Muscle

A small muscle inside the eye that controls the shape of the lens to help focus light onto the retina during accommodation.

Computer Vision Syndrome (CVS)

Also known as digital eye strain, it is a group of eye

and vision-related problems resulting from prolonged computer and screen use.

Digital Eye Strain

Symptoms including eye discomfort, headaches, and blurred vision caused by prolonged use of digital devices such as computers, tablets, and smartphones.

Ergonomics

The study of people's efficiency in their working environment, particularly how the setup of one's workspace can reduce strain and improve comfort, including eye comfort.

Hyperopia

A vision condition, also known as farsightedness, where distant objects are seen more clearly than near objects due to the light entering the eye focusing behind the retina.

Myopia

A vision condition, also known as nearsightedness, where near objects are seen more clearly than distant objects due to the light entering the eye focusing in front of the retina.

Presbyopia

An age-related condition where the eye's lens loses its flexibility, making it difficult to focus on close objects.

Retina

The light-sensitive layer at the back of the eye that converts light into neural signals sent to the brain for visual recognition.

Screen Time

The amount of time spent using devices with screens such as computers, smartphones, and tablets.

Vergence

The simultaneous movement of both eyes in opposite directions to obtain or maintain single binocular vision.

Virtual Reality (VR)

A simulated experience created by using VR headsets that can replicate real or imagined environments and interactions.

Wearable Technology

Electronic devices worn on the body, such as smart glasses or contact lenses with digital displays, which can impact eye health.

20-20-20 Rule

A guideline to reduce eye strain by taking a 20-second break to look at something 20 feet away every 20 minutes of screen time.

Glare

Bright light that interferes with vision and can cause discomfort, often from screens or overhead lights.

Optic Nerve

The nerve that transmits visual information from the retina to the brain.

Photochromic Technology

Lens technology that darkens in response to sunlight and helps protect the eyes from UV rays.

Cataract

A clouding of the lens in the eye leading to a decrease in vision, often associated with aging.

Age-Related Macular Degeneration (AMD)

A medical condition which may result in blurred or no vision in the center of the visual field, typically occurring in older adults.

Chapter 11

Resources & References

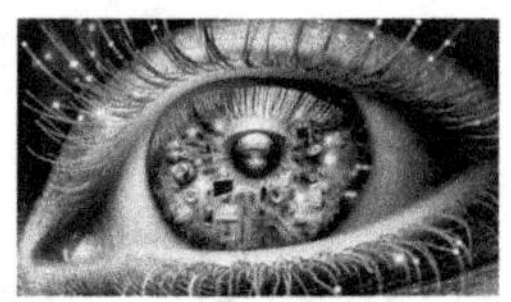

American Optometric Association (AOA)

Website: aoa.org

The AOA offers comprehensive resources on eye health, including guidelines on digital eye strain, blue light exposure, and tips for maintaining healthy vision.

American Academy of Ophthalmology (AAO)

Website: aao.org

The AAO provides educational materials, research articles, and updates on the latest advancements in ophthalmology and eye care.

National Eye Institute (NEI)

Website: nei.nih.gov

Part of the National Institutes of Health, the NEI conducts and supports research on eye diseases and vision disorders. Their website offers valuable information on a wide range of eye health topics.

Mayo Clinic – Eye Health

Website: mayoclinic.org/eye-health

Mayo Clinic provides expert advice and research-backed information on eye conditions, treatments, and preventive measures to maintain good eye health.

Harvard Health Publishing – Vision and Eye Health

Website: health.harvard.edu/topics/vision-and-eye-health

Harvard Health offers articles and resources on various eye health topics, including tips for reducing digital eye strain and the impact of blue light on vision.

American Academy of Optometry (AAOpt)

Website: aaopt.org

The AAOpt focuses on promoting the art and science of vision care through lifelong learning. It offers resources for both professionals and the public on maintaining optimal eye health.

EyeCare America

Website: eyecareamerica.org

A public service program of the American Academy of Ophthalmology, EyeCare America provides eye health information and access to eye care services.

Vision Council – Digital Eye Strain Report

Website: thevisioncouncil.org

The Vision Council's report on digital eye strain offers insights into the prevalence of digital eye strain, its symptoms, and recommended solutions.

Ophthalmology Times

Website: ophthalmologytimes.com

A professional publication that covers the latest research, trends, and news in ophthalmology and vision care, providing valuable insights for both professionals and the public.

About Dr. Martinelli

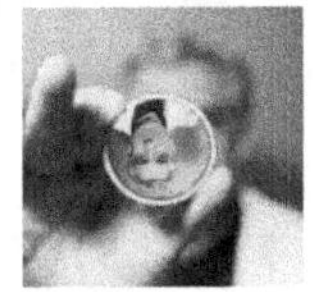

With 27 years as an optometric physician on the front lines prior to earning his medical degree, Dr. Martinelli now brings more than 35 years of private practice experience, combined with medicine, providing rare insight and guidance with respect to patient care philosophy.

Dr. Martinelli is a graduate of St. George's University School of Medicine, Pennsylvania College of Optometry, as well as Washington & Jefferson College. He is a physician member of the American Medical Association (AMA), Fellow of the American Academy of Optometry (FAAO), and the American Optometric Association (AOA).

His clinical articles have been featured over the years in various publications, and he also very much enjoys teaching, with more than a decade mentoring countless students as a preceptor in ocular disease for the Pennsylvania College of Optometry.

Dr. Martinelli has spoken for Alcon and Allergan, as well as nationally and internationally with topics involving medical eye care, glaucoma, and refractive surgery such as LASIK.

Also by Dr. Martinelli

Books:

Vision & Neurology Casebook: Real-World Insights for Primary Eye Care & Family Medicine

Labs & Imaging for Primary Eye Care

Substack:

The Fine Art of Patient Management